S0-BAK-044

THE PEAR ORCHARD

JOANNE WEBER

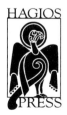

HAGIOS
PRESS

Copyright © 2007 Joanne Weber

All rights reserved. No part of this publication may be reproduced, stored in a retrieval system, or transmitted in any form or by any means without the prior written permission of the publisher or by licensed agreement with Access: The Canadian Copyright Licensing Agency. Exceptions will be made in the case of a reviewer, who may quote brief passages in a review to print in a magazine or newspaper, broadcast on radio or television, or post on the Internet.

Library and Archives Canada Cataloguing in Publication

Weber, Joanne, 1959-
 The pear orchard / Joanne Weber.

Poems.
ISBN 978-0-9739727-7-1

 I. Title.
PS8645.E23P42 2007   C811'.6   C2007-901948-X

Edited by Paul Wilson.
Designed and typeset by Donald Ward.
Cover painting: *A Couple of Pears 2* by Karen Yurkovich.
Cover design by Yves Noblet.
Set in Adobe Caslon Pro and Trajan Pro.
Printed and bound in Canada at Houghton Boston Printers
& Lithographers, Saskatoon.

The publishers gratefully acknowledge the assistance of the Saskatchewan Arts Board, The Canada Council for the Arts, and the Cultural Industries Development Fund (Saskatchewan Department of Culture, Youth & Recreation) in the production of this book.

HAGIOS PRESS
Box 33024 Cathedral PO
Regina SK   S4T 7X2

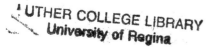
LUTHER COLLEGE LIBRARY
University of Regina

For my parents, Edward and Lois Weber,
who led me to the first word.

Contents

Advent

The Fields

A Deaf Woman in the Orchard

Inside a deaf woman, a pear orchard grows.
As a child, she whirls among mirrors and pears,
her finger tips brush the blue black branches,
her gown is sheathed in the raiment of broken lights
splashing over green, red and golden fruit.
She sits in the darkness, waiting for someone to call her
from the orchard.

Yet she takes her place in the world,
has a body, a body like everyone else's. Her mother says,
the lights are only flashes, fragments leading
to half formed ideas, a sudden brilliance swallowed by darkness.
Yet broken lights are better than silence.

At least they ward off boredom,
you can play with them in your mind,
look at the trees spangled with hanging mirrors,
such loveliness should compensate for the pears
that cannot be eaten, you'll never fully grasp their meaning,
their enunciation, their place in conversing or even in books.

Her mother tells her, be satisfied with shimmering lights,
think of them as fairies flying among the trees,
for the fruit of the orchard, my dear,
was never meant for you.

THE CHRISTMAS PEAR

To our bodies turn we then, that so
    Weak men on love revealed may look;
Love's mysteries in souls do grow,
    But yet the body is his book.

John Donne
"The Ecstasy"

The Lie

In twelfth century France,
a deaf woman and a hearing man are laid to rest
in an iron sarcophagus, she on top of him.
Their faces become two masks
snapped together, her headdress
of pears covers his helmet,
his eyes are embedded in her forehead,
the man's lips pressed
under his wife's open mouth.

This is the way he likes it,
a language of touch
for the deaf and dumb.
She nods in agreement,
lies in their cool tomb, her body
a misplaced cipher in both languages.

Christmas Pear I

On Christmas morning, I walk backwards
three times around a tree heavy with pears,
peer into the thicket, trying to make out the face
of my future beloved.

Silly girls giggle as I search out the heart of the pear tree,
beginning to fear that none of this was true,
that I would find my body cast in a pear,
letting flesh enter this heavy bottomed fruit,
becoming the bellowed skirt, the swollen belly.

I pray, don't let my body be
the only true thing about love
on Christmas morning.

Geertgen Tot Sint Jans: The Holy Kinship

In this pear orchard, my elongated head
is an egg wrapped in a green turban.
Over a golden net of diamonds and pearls,
sectioned by rubies and sapphires,
bordered by pearls, fringed by miniature golden leaves,

a shining arch runs to the apex of the turban
a ruby telling the point.

The mummied egg has a wimple yet,
the white linen falling down my neck,
the hills of my amber gown hides
my spreading buttocks.

I saw you last night, stealing the pears
from my father's garden, there
you bit into the green and bitter fruit,
threw them against the stone wall.

I can't move the mummied egg
any further out the window, to call out to you,
to warn you of the consequences
in my father's house
especially if we are to marry.

Surely afterwards, the egg won't break
when you tap on my eyes.

Seduction

Remove your wimple, let us be soft
as I reach around you. Your womb
swells against my hand against the wall
of the sarcophagus, your breath pushing your rib cage
into my chest. Your broken words throb
in my ear, let my language come between us,
hard as a young green pear.

Christmas Pear II

Was I not a virgin in these dark nights?
I didn't see your face through the Christmas tree.
Instead I walked beside my mother, holding my prayer book,
rosary entwined between my fingers.

There were pots and pans in the kitchen,
the hem of my amber dress needed to be mended,
my wimple askew, the jewels heavy.
I was to learn to play the lute.

In the warm light of candles,
I turned my face when you lifted
my amber dress, hoping I would be deceived.

How could this be done to me?

Jan Van Eyck: Giovanni Arnolfini and His Bride

Hastily you climb down
from our marriage bed in the late afternoon
and struggle into the pompous velvets and brocaded silks.
The stays must be fastened right.
Your wimple is to be laid aside after this day.
You are a noblewoman now, soon to be fitted
in a stiff headdress of pears,

in this bedroom of your mother's weavings,
dark furniture and opaque windows.

Soon they'll appear
to sign some contract or other
concerning cloth? Glass? Cows? Chickens?

Your brandy pup plays at our feet
as the octagonal mirror framed in walnut
reflects the entry of the burghers.
They come in the midst of our passion
most holy. You are round with our child.
Your eyes burn, you give it away
by holding my hand and you wait with guilt.

They say to our white faces,
You are so young. Later you ask,
Why are you so obsequious to these burghers
when you should be eager for my love?

Your eyes burn.

Sylva

Husband, could you not come home?
The bolts of silk, velvets, brocades from Tuscany
always come through your messengers.
Impatiently I throw your notes to the ground.
They cannot have been written by you,
these stilted declarations of love.

I wait, with oh so much longing,
it sickens my bones. You must see
how great is my womb, the pear
protruding from the cage of my hips
with each passing day.

The Spell

Two of us are in this cold stone tomb
rattling our breath, trying to form words
that would break the lid over us.

You lay on top of me,
arching backwards to make room for the child,
crushing me with your weight,

your eyes unblinking
under that fantastic headdress
of pears, no tears on your stone face
pocked by rain, while the child's cries
will not break the spell between us,
trapping us forever under the lid.

Christmas Pear III

You are away when our child is born.
Tonight, she stands with me on her tiptoes,
lighting the Advent wreath. I keep her away
from the tree in the great hall, she is too young
to know her true love. I peer
through the black and bare branches,
well below to the tree stump immersed
in a basin of water and up to the angel above me.
I dare not look straight ahead.

Chartres

In the building of Chartres, may only the deaf man be a saint?
His bones and sinews force up the dank stones, his fingers grip
the impossible corners, grope for the hairline crevices.

Away from him, behind stone walls my hands form signs
in dark rooms, our daughter learning by candlelight.
In the chapel, I cannot sway as easily through the stations,
this pear headdress is too cumbersome.

And the master builder, my husband, is always away in Tuscany,
I am anxious over the hunched backs of the wretched men
further up the scaffolding. The deaf man knows only
pulling, balancing, and lifting stone onto a wall.
I see his nausea, the filth of his clay-soaked rags,
and the blood racing the blue veins, the tiny rivers of his hands.

The men wander to their homes in the mist,
my troubadours sing to them of their purpose,
singing from under the cover of trees
while the deaf man stands silently.

Propping my pear headdress against the back of my chair,
I could love him, those fingers so strong, agile.

Instead, I pull a ring from my finger,
studded with brilliant rubies, emeralds, sapphires,
throw it at his feet, a plea to go on,

or to leave here, and take with him,
the darkness of blood on stone.

Chastisement

Enough woman, about my raiding that pear orchard.
So what if I had no motive other than the pleasure of stealing?
It was a childish prank, a foolish frolic with young boys.

You were not even hungry,
coming back from a feast, where you snitched
the roast duck in your father's kitchen,
choking on the bones behind the table of pastries
in the smoky room, until the cook chased you out.

Dressed in silks with a leather pouch full of gold,
you had no need of money or anything to sell.
You had friends just as foolish as you,
bored hours ago with the troubadours.

Enough woman, you don't need to go on and on
about a boyhood story I should have never told you.
You talk too much, flapping your hands
like a crazy goose, honking and hissing.

You smashed the fruit against the stone wall,
you ought to have wanted a pear
that would run down your chin,
one that would have reminded you of me,
just one.

Do you hear me? I leave tomorrow for Tuscany again.

Book of Hours

My expectations are too high, it's right for you to go,
flee the briars, escape the borders of my life

so that I may chant these days, these hours,
sleep these nights alone, I may find courage

to invoke these saints, praise their lives,
beckon their mother, pray for grace,

for courage
to flee these briars, escape these borders,
to chant new hours, new joy.

Return

Husband, welcome home.
You must be tired after such a long journey.
I'll have Jacques take the horses to the stable,
come warm yourself before the great fire,
oh your hands are so stiff with the cold,
your fingers bend like wiry twine.
I shall come to you later this evening,
when you are warm again.

Here is a pear to stay your hunger,
as we wake slowly to the silence,
learn its nouns, parse its verbs,
the whorls of silence will be laid down

while you wait for me, let the juice of the pear
trickle slowly down your chin
as you bite into my vanilla flesh.

When you roll the seeds under your tongue,
I will become yours again.

Annunciation

When did he lightly turn to me, a blue angel,
swinging a thurible, clouds of incense around me?
Or is it a stork legged lily? I'm not sure,
at Mass nothing much happens
except for incense, the smell of heaven.

Later that afternoon, I understand
that it was only the milky light from the stained glass window,
high in the nave, the same light coming
over the high casement in our home,
my hands drop the amber thread for the tear in my dress,
I pull the pear headdress from my aching head.

The blue angel puts a finger to his lips while gold shines all around.
Let all mortal flesh keep silence.

How is another child possible? I've borne a daughter
(is it not enough?) to a man who is always away.
I've worn my pear headdress faithfully (it is so heavy these days).
Angel, how can you steep yourself in my womb, float in the tea
of menstrual blood, broken leaves, torn flowers and smashed fruit?

Let all mortal flesh keep silence.

The hand slides behind my back, lifting me up. Oh lifting me up.
I've forgotten everything. Oh, let it be done to me.

Rembrandt's Pears

Gossamer filaments wrap around
the pears nestled against apples,
the threads perhaps leftover from rain,
stretching in the light, a delicacy suggesting
a smallness, a seed
growing somewhere, I don't know
what Rembrandt knows about pears,
about the brown seed growing
within my alabaster flesh.

I know that an orchard was raided,
bruised and slashed pears
were heaped in a cart,
driven off in the night
for no reason at all.

Although the orchard raid is a smallness, a seed
that will grow no further in us,
what Rembrandt knows is in me,
is enough for the new pear tree.

Christmas Pear IV

On Christmas eve, the pear tree is glowing
through the black wizened branches,
its fingers scratching the warm golden light
of lit advent candles.

On this silent night, no cry echoes in the darkness,
the warm heavy fruit now houses a sleeping child.
All around her is decay, the golden translucent skin of the pear
is mottled with black cuts, sprays of spores, and ripening orange.

Still the child sleeps.
I caution the silly girls not to wake
the child warm and flushed under the membrane

less she come out too soon.
Sound in the world is not to be unloosed

until the child wakes,
caged between my ballooning hips.
I want this true love on Christmas morn.
I want this to be done to me.

The Pear Orchard

Mother, now that you've let me be deaf,
scraped your womb of its dank winter trees,
cleared the unkempt patches,
you've let me be a pure seed begun
in you, a room of buried longings.

Your passion sang long and hard for me,
this lushness beginning in the spring orchard.

My longings begin their fleshly protrusions,
my most wild need is heard
and is not yours, but mine

as the dream of pears accompanies me
through your seasons until the burst

of my deaf body, a blossom
through your floor, my limbs, strong green vines
push through your windows, straining
with the flesh of my stray desire:

Let me be deaf, hold my ear to your breast,
let me see how the pear orchard grows.

THE BLACK POND

For I am every dead thing,
In whom Love wrought new alchemy.

John Donne
"A Nocturnal Upon St. Lucy's Day"

Chatelaine

It would help things if you were more with it,
consult the seven habits of highly effective people,
instead of hagiography, your book of medieval saints,
sewing golden velvet and brocade dresses,
I like you in jeans now that it is harvest.

If you'd pack my lunch, drive out to the field,
speak of the small things, if you'd leave the soup simmering,
drive to the nearest town, with the labeled part under your arm
while I wait, drinking coffee in the truck.

At midnight I come home, covered in grain dust,
you are still up, canning jars cooling on the table,
the pages of a book of saints fanning in the open window.
You don't even look at me, you want to be a chatelaine,
would lock me in the cellar, among the tubers,
tomatoes, crab apples and beets.

I'd hear your footsteps overhead, the boards creaking,
as you jangle the keys.

St. Augustine

Augustine's original sin begins
in a dusty African town, his sandals
slap on sun-baked clay, his voice atop
the whooping of his friends as they climb the cold stone wall.

Only moss softens their grip on the crevices,
absorbs the blood running down their fingers
as they rip the soft and mouldy fruit,
shredding leaves and branches.

The gardener has counted these pears
toward his yearly harvest,
dreaming of amber wine through which the sun
would send mirrored flecks of light.

Augustine and his friends spit creamed gobs of fruit,
as they run the rickety cart alongside the stone wall,
spill a new road of pears, a cobbled walk,
where their sandals cut black crevices,
a grout beginning its decay inwards.

The Black Pond

Your back is turned as I peer over the open book,
on the table underneath the kitchen window,
the pages fluttering like birds in the night.
The autumn wind has come in with me
but you do not turn to the open door, you are counting
canning jars now heavy with red, amber and green fruit.

You forget there is a black pond in
in this pear orchard.
The picture doesn't show it,
a pool of melted jet lapping quietly
against coal heaped shores
lined by pear trees, their fruit
caught in the black crackling light.

Round mirrors spin slowly on the branches,
catching amber, russet, green, silver and gold
patches on pears twirling heavy and low
while the green black leaves titter.

Do not startle as you always do
as I approach you from behind.
My hands interlock below your breasts
while the moonlight sends the mirrors
and pears a jangling in our faces.

Temptation in the Garden

Come with me,
leave the holy books,
the silence of icons, the honeyed flesh
of saints, spit out the creamy pulp
of their words and the hard brown seeds.

Take my hand, come with me
Lavender's blue, dilly, dilly,
Lavender's green, when I am king,
Dilly, dilly, you shall be queen.

When we are finally out of our orchard,
we can look over our shoulders
at the reflection of the black pond,
the spinning mirrored lights and golden orbs
will sing together like morning stars
of our new love, your body
round in the hip, full in the belly,
your heavy breasts pushing up against me.

I will take any fruit, even a pear
already bitten by your even white teeth,
I'll catch your seeds on my tongue

so I will not be alone.
Come away, come.

Artifacts

I am tempted to see you again,
but before your coming,
I pray for an artifact
from the isle of Crete. The jar or its shards
is for my cherishing, my honouring

on a page of Kells, studded with jewels,
bordered by a serene blue from crushed lapis lazuli

while I stand in an open tent, disdainful
receiving pearls from a timid serving maid
while mad dogs and wild boars
circle me in the tapestry
of my apprehension.

Shall I lose my obsession with the jar, page, tapestry
when you come again?

Simple Gifts I

While we wait out this darkness,
the turning mirrors incessantly blink
in our eyes, oh, think of me as your king,
a medieval metaphor surely pleases you.

Think of me too, as a simple man,
I enjoy simple pleasures:
a walk in my fields each day,
measuring the stubble with the toe of my boot.

These November stalks are what's left
in the wind of a threatened harvest,
a simple vocabulary, mine is one
of crops and the weather, a concentration
of nouns, verbs, and adjectives
that explain how I got from the farmhouse
to the barn, to feed the cattle,
to chop the barley and to fill the silos.

This plain language should lead us out of the orchard
where the crowns are heavy on our heads.
You, in your amber gown, are mesmerized
by the evening beginning its violet wash atop
of the green black trees, corduroyed trunks
of the trees backlit by a darkening blue
descending upon the glitter of coal black shores.

I must explain these things very carefully
less the mirrors turn forever.

The Odyssey

The crying wakes me in the Aegean morning.
I quickly offer flowers
and bathing perfumes stored in stone jars
by rocks on the shore.

Circe's eyes follow, and the howl of sirens
dog my scurrying steps down garden paths,
through chambers, kitchens, baths and closets.

Closets.
The sheets of Odysseus.
The sheets that wrapped, bound
and billowed with each breath
hid him,
hid him
from the Aegean morning and its poets,
from water bearers and shepherds,
from washerwomen and lepers.

The pear tree that forms the canopy over us,
keeps our bed intact, my wits weave
the work of days and hands
into a virgin's girdle for my body
thickening with age.

I walk
in the Aegean morning with its poets,
water bearers and shepherds,
washerwomen and lepers,
waiting.

The Holy

What is it about Odysseus?
I am your king here in this orchard,
your body beats against mine,
against these imaginary lives,
these flashing bits of light
leaving dead patches and wilted leaves
among the branches of the pear trees.

But holy things are for the holy.

The body is holy, your deaf body
is the pear, its flesh cushions
our bodies in perpetual embrace
in the waters of the black pond churning
bile, excrement, urine, your menstrual blood.

From these waters, pears grow heavy and round,
promising a harvest of preserves, jam and wine,
or juice trickling down the chin,
juice from the core.

Boadicea

I am raw in winter
with blue etched cheeks and coarse mane
blown back by war.

I plan destruction of the Romans
who raped my daughters before my fire
though I will not win.

My men in winter
are simple living in a forest,
our gods are in trees. The rains chill
and they warm themselves
on my fire.

I will sacrifice my fire
to the rains though I am tired
living for winter men. My Celtic blood
makes me too fierce when
I ride into the Roman camp at night.

With my dead men at my feet,
my Roman masters chilled by the rains,
there will be no men of winter at my fire.

I am large for men of summer.

Syphilis

Boadicea or whoever you are at the moment,
your longing for a perfect body
will become a syphilis, will smirch your fruit.
The madness will etch itself into your warm flesh,
lines that blacken, curl inwards, your flesh
will become brown in the narrow troughs.

Under the flashing lights among the dark trees,
golden and russet orbs spinning into the night,
I smear the silver salve, mercury
over your breasts and belly.

Is my warning not sufficient?
The mercurial quicksilver flashes
life death life death
You must choose your deaf body.
It is really that simple.

Simone Weil

My mother hid new nylons
in my drawers, while I
the trolless Simone, the red virgin
rose from the communist sea.

My roommates cooked me
expensive cuts of meat,
while I paid no attention,
paying for a maid
who never existed.

I formed trade unions, ate cold potatoes,
taught philosophy and Alain was delighted.

But this was not bravado,
I really thought this way,
with imperfect knowledge, I took love
with no apology to you.

Catherine Earnshaw

Now, you say you are Heathcliff.
Believe what you will, say no more
except that a Jacobean angel attacks
you on your Sunday tramp through the moor.

Hey woman, your hair is caught by thistles
as you flail in the rain for hours.
Inevitably, you are thrown into the mud.

The wind has died, the rain is slowing.
Get up. The angel is waiting.
Get up. It is your blood.

Isolde the Fair to Evelyn Waugh (*Brideshead Revisited*)

With cloak random and wild,
I, Isolde the Fair rage
at the threshold of Brideshead.

I demand allegiance from Waugh, an English sot
for I am the soul of the world,
all eyes on the western front
watch my billowing cloak.

Waugh gives me Charles Ryder,
and I strike him with the star of passion.
The rays are harp strings; each note tells mercy
on his blessed face. The ethereal world
folds in around him like a heavily scented harem,
for the gillyflowers are in bloom.

To Waugh, I rage.
O artist, passion is my life. You thwart Charles.
I am born into a Catholic family, settled
into boredom. Their ethereal religion folds
around me like a heavily scented harem
for martyrdom is in bloom.

I am Charles! The ghost of his woman.
Where shall I go?

My cloak, see what you've made of it.
A sea at storm, each line you create
fills my mouth with salt water.

Where shall I go?

(As Tristan lay dying, my heart soared.
I meant to conquer the western world
with passion. My cloak, random and wild
brought the sea at storm to Tristan's corpse).

And you took me, artist,
took my soul to the world.
To Brideshead.
I rage.

Ezekial 16

I would like to think
my love made a difference to you,
as you lay in your blood.

I am your king.
I clothed you with lace from Ghent,
wool warm from Flemish looms.
I heard you singing,
the wine of your voice warmed
my gut for many years
and I was king
only because of your happiness.

When your sadness returns,
I heap the rubies and sapphires on your head,
let them rain down your white wimple
as you peer out the casement
down at the pear orchard.

You don't even notice
the jewels at your feet
while you remain in the house
of my love, lying in your blood.

Fanny Mendelssohn: A Letter to Felix

We were children
when you chased me up the staircase
with a butcher knife.
My feet struck sparks on the stairs
before I flew into the closet,
quickly closing the latch.

My cloistered years in our Berlin home
had me dancing in the piano room.
The windows were thrown open
to the flowers on the terrace.
I kissed your portrait and lamented
your departing to Paris or London.

My cloistered years had me waiting.
I fingered secretly your music scores,
delighting to find my songs among your own.

Now you discover me with your music.
You tell me to fly.
Your words strike sparks
quick as my feet on the stairs.

Hours later, you find me sobbing
in the dark closet
and through the bouquet of wilted flowers
clutched in your moist hand,
I grow older.

Anger

Your anger at your deafness has split our voice,
sliced it evenly as a pear in half,
the white fruit moist and quivering,
glistening brown seeds lay
helplessly for the scattering

as it falls among damp newspaper,
potato peelings, and candy wrappers
in the kitchen garbage.

In this orchard, we swim in the putrid black waters,
push away the slimy fronds,
of discarded newspaper and plastic
netted between our fingers.
Afterwards we lean against the corduroyed trees,
blinking under a canopy of pears and mirrors.

Are the fields not better,
a wild and windy place where the Russian thistle blows,
where my combine splits the stem from the seed,
the chaff blowing up and away from us.

Marie Curie

Pierre. Quick.
Destruction divorces sun and moon
and Renoir sends his regrets.
His ballerinas are still preparing
for the stage and I go down,
slippers in one hand
when the lights catch me,

you roar. I shrink in my brilliance
you are red faced, having carried
our bicycles up to our flat.
I hear you. The wheels scrape
against the door frames in the stairwells.

Pierre, I have it.
The sun and moon reign in separate spheres
and begin their journey toward each other
only when I go slowly into the dance.

But you tease me, pulling the flower
from your buttonhole.
I take your hand and start
for our laboratory in the attic.
Wait, you say. You want to go slowly,
shall we have tea? You smile,
it is spring, the mud puddles
are full of children.

But shining rings are waiting
in the attic for our discovery.

You pretend to wither.
I have it. Pierre!
My robe is too lovely
to wear for only five minutes,
the flowers are too sweet, too young,
who am I to tell the sun and moon
to marry again in a twinkling
when upon the centuries
I must dance?

You roar.

Simple Gifts II

Look, I am a simple man.
Never have I wanted refinement, portraits, and philosophy.
Instead I truck the wheat, dump it in an elevator,
leaving it to others to sell.
At noon, I eat the sandwiches in my pail
at the back of the truck,
small animals skitter past my feet
and the swallows in the sky
sing to me.

The harvest is the antidote to your strange anguish,
whether you are deaf or not matters
little to others. You are not satisfied

but one day, you'll slip away behind me.
Thinking all is clear, I'll back over you,
slice your arm or a hand. You'll be hurt
more if I don't signal to you.

My simple gifts include
the field, fallow and folded with winter wheat,
my love for you is in the combine skulking behind the silo.

It is just that, no more.

Augustine's Pear

> Late have I loved You, beauty so ancient yet so new.
> St. Augustine
> *Confessions*

In the night, Augustine raided a pear orchard with his friends.
Afterwards, the pear hung around his neck,
a heavy bottomed millstone,
a golden belly besmirched,
his soul blackened with knowledge

of pears stolen for no reason at all
except for the sake of easy camaraderie
with the other boys. Loneliness

made him into a bishop, a deafness
louder than the cries of his concubine,
the hawking in the dusty marketplace,
the chatter of monkeys, the bellow of elephants,
the tinkle of gold, silence is now a pear

ripe for the taking.

Noise

Your hands are noisy when our child is conceived.
They rush to play a violin, an old tune
that your mother taught you during winter evenings
on the farm, they rush to whittle a stick, polish a pear,
crank a wrench out in the tool shed.

Your hands travel up and down my body,
a desperate fiddle as Nero once played
before the burning of Rome, now Carthage
is a holy fire, sizzling with wild and stray desires

during which our hands should weave
through the silent flames.

Renoir: On the Terrace

Soon there will be two vulnerable women in this orchard,
a small girl shadowed by her mother,
the rain streaking a faint flush on her cheeks,
her hair, a brown field for the brave red blossoms
pointing to her eyes. No delicacy is possible

without her mother imitating her, the lips, the flush,
the hair, the posies crowding round her
scarred eyes. She is cautious.
Why does she live here?

The lips, the flush, the hair,
the posies crowding around her become
a union of caution and innocence,
scars and rain.

Lara: To Zhivago

You go down on Ash Wednesday
to pray to me, an icon.
Avoiding my face, you reach
beneath my robes
for the sun rising behind my crown.

You know me.
Across the steppes, the wind lashes
you with my name.
We sit in a winter chair
drawn by irate saints
across mosaic stones.

We laugh, you look down
into the booth of my furs
combed by the wind
as you whip the saints
past Eastern cathedrals,
onion roofs announcing Lent.

My face is dissolving in our shame.
In the wind, the mosaic promises
gravel for the raven's crop.

Let it be summer then,
saints are stones skipping to me on water,
bringing me your silence: our praise
as Lent rides the wind.

Please go down on Ash Wednesday,
restore us, restore your icon.
Behind these onion roofs,
the rising sun is ours.

The Source of Light

Ah, this is the source of light
in this orchard, the cubed lights
flickering over the black pool,
ricocheting between mirrors,
pears and the dark green leaves.

This is where your desire comes from,
like any young woman, you want a body
that is not yours, in which deafness is irrelevant.

This is where your life comes from,
flitting from portrait to portrait,
frame to frame in this gallery

of famous people long ago on the Aegean,
in the Flemish lowlands, the British isles
who have found certain truths
which flash brilliantly in the dark
speaking of all things but you.

Karensgaard

I.

After pleading for a lighter burden,
I slam my love down on a marble slab
somewhere in the woods.

Home again, I light a candle,
lie with the dead child on my bed.

In the next room, friends sing.
Their song is deep cinnamon,
their strings, dark honey, a mother's voice.

It is too sweet. I offer the child a breast.
She cannot suck.

II.

Water invades my home. The sun shines through
the windows, on the water standing in the rooms.
My poems are lily pads afraid to shoot a stem.

There is mould and I can not set my house in order.
The walls rot.

My friends and I stand on the foundation,
try to build a fire.

I build the child into a crude grave
with stones from the fireplace.
The gravestone repairs a corner of the foundation.
We are a tribe, a race, my friends and I.

Our song is like cinnamon, strings of honey
in a mother's voice.

I must sleep.

III.

Karensgaard stands now.
Apple and pear trees give me fruit
to sweeten with cinnamon and dark honey.
The cream from scrubbed barns stays my hunger.
On late October afternoons,
bonfires and roasted chestnuts
in the clear cold air beckon children
from the wide mountain valley.
My voice reaches the horses in the pasture,
my man halts his plough.

After dark at Karensgaard,
leaves rap at our door. The moon shines
through the window on copper pans in the kitchen
and between sheets and caresses
in the high quilted bed,
I see the return of the child.

George Sand

Under the piano I lay in the late hours of the afternoon,
my dress drawn up around my knees,
my fingers laced over my swollen belly,
the windows opened wide to the lengthening shadows.

I would have worn pants but none would fit today,
now the ladies will smirk and say, you cannot deny
your feminity, nevertheless my dress is drawn to my knees.
I feel the breeze tickle my inner thighs,
set the petticoats rustling and I reach in,
pressing carefully my protruding navel.

Oh Chopin, my love thundering above me,
will you ever be exquisite in any other way,
your long white fingers
pressing the notes ever so lightly,
pretending that there is no child between us?

Woman's Hair

Look, I promise you nothing about the child,
not until you have a body, warm, deaf
not until you can praise your wide hips,
and the belly I used to warm with the flat of my hand
in the mornings before the night stole away from our bed.
Remember before I went out into the fields,
remember how I'd tell you, the silken dirt beneath my feet
is that of a woman's hair?

Héloïse

The October morning waits for the sun
to cloak the cloister wall. How you gag
at this shriving, your hands twist
on the Holy Writ. The black robes keep
your body back from the altar: the sacrament
you refuse. You weep in a wimple teased by wind.
You know he is a motherless child. You make him
master while you live with women.
You lie festering,
his glory sprung from your cell.

Teresa of Avila

Never mind him, you are now with child,
go lie down if you're tired, eat steak if your blood is low.
I catch her napping through the Spanish grille,
her prayer book falling to the floor.

In the garden, she has an orgasm in the embrace of our Lord.
She tells me to be quiet about it. Read my spiritual diary,
she says, thirteen years of silence until in one dry season
he slides his hand behind my back,
lifting me up, oh lifting me up.

She clacks her rosary fiercely,
admonishing in a thick Spanish tongue,
eat steak if your blood is low,
go lie down if you're tired.

Pieta

I.

Act quickly under the winter moon,
instruct me with image, give me confidence
so that in Jerusalem, I may become
worthy of you.

II.

You send me to swans trapped
in old women, their wombs dry,
their sons dead, each woman mourning
on her private throne in the Sistine.

In the streets, mandolins strain
faint notes into a canticle
while I pray with the women
on the feast of martyrs.

You ring bells over the old women.
I watch your seeded air transform them into
swans erupting through bone, skin and skull,
warm and bloody under the winter moon.

III.

From your scaffolding, you send me, an ant running
through the labyrinth of paint pots and statues
to fetch your crucifix from above your bed
for you need inspiration.

I must go into the dark street, speak to no one.
I must be furtive though my way is clear.
I must take no shawl or purse, no food for beggars,

pray not to be deceived by beauty in the fires
or by men forming strained canticles.

Have I sorted our seeds for this moment?
Or do you mock me?

IV.

I knock: no answer but a crucifix over your bed.
You, my beloved, do not await me here.

Yet, in these streets, you shoot enthusiasm
into me. From your seeds I find one,
our son in making. My womb in winter
is a queen busy in choosing a suitor.

V.

The winter ushers in the feast of martyrs.
Every saint prophesies the abortion,
our unborn child cut out and your severed head
placed over me under the winter moon.
I have chosen your seed and your head.

VI.

Baptist! Can you speak?

VII.

While I walk through winter,
fires catch the notes of the canticle,
the seeded air gives you back to me.

VIII.

I meditate on your wounds.

IX.

In Jerusalem, I hold you, pieta.
I am a throne of comfort,
a swan settling under the moon's triumph,
a winter's tale, a myth retold.
You ring bells over me, your canticle is seeded air.
You lie over my womb, a medium for men.

Héloïse: White Martyrdom

In your white martyrdom
        love is strange. That kind of shining
has an enamel finish. The exact intensity
        of milkiness and sheen,
the seed pearls of your cap,
        the cream at Abelard's home in Brittany,
the new child in a white shift for the morning feedings
        wait in radiance.

ADVENT

I wonder, by my troth, what thou and I
Did, till we loved?

John Donne
"The Good Morrow"

At that time Mary got ready and hurried to
a town in the hill country of Judea, where
she entered Zechariah's home and greeted
Elizabeth.

Luke 1:39

Dorothy Day: Annunciation

I liked myself better
before I became a saint, those hours
of picking at the bedcovers while he slept.

Wandering in his shed, through rows
of his specimens, the biologist's world
of splendors, my passion howls for him

down through the kitchen, pots and their lids,
the stacks of plates and porcelain bowls
rattling in their fury under my tormented breath.

I batten down the hatches, ride out the storm once more,
my belief in God the Father, God the Son,
and God the Holy Spirit will soon dissipate,
become a womanish obsession again.

I glance sideways at him in our bed, still he sleeps
and the long loneliness goes on,

and on until the angel comes,
a blue angel swinging a thurible,
holding his finger to my lips,
the horn of the lily fitting tightly over my ear.

In our bed, I tell him of the angel,
how I am with child. He stirs and wakes,
tells me, well, you heard wrong, you are only thinking
of the angel in some art collection
probably an illuminated manuscript,
the longings of man put down,
translated into myth.

My man falls asleep again.
I take our daughter down the road
to a friend. From far away,
he shudders as he turns in his sleep.

Advent

This is a new season, the dank winter trees
drip in frosted rain. In the fog I feel
for your white neck that should lift up
like a swan banked in a snow,
you are not here.

Your breasts no longer press
against me, your soft thigh no longer rolls over my hip.
Even the smell of your menstrual blood is gone.
I stoop by the black pool and my hand trails through cold water
catching filmy fronds of algae.

Shivering by this black pond,
I try to remember the sky dipping low
to harvested fields, every stalk jack frozen,
corrugated black lumps that were once your silken hair
soon to be adorned with pearls of snow.

Silence

She has left me in this orchard,
I slap the black waters, hoping to see a ripple
out from the coal heaped shores. I hear nothing.
I can't even smell the pears I know to be hanging
from the branches of the dead trees.

She's gone to Elizabeth down the road,
old Zechariah must watch them talking
with a morose eye now stricken
silent with winter snow,
the ice speckled fields lie barren,
barricaded by bare caragana hedges,
the sodden lumps of earth wait for a hand

to turn things over to the spring. If I get there,
I'll buy a tractor part off the old farmer,
he'd appreciate some business,
him being struck dumb,
making ridiculous signs with his hands,
his wife fat with his child.

I slap the black waters again.
Who'd want a child at that age?

Elizabeth's Advice

Silly women think your words are eloquent,
floating out to the world on soft downy feathers,
they love your metaphors.
They are so full of feeling.

Women, young and old,
get together in a gaggle, bite into unripe pears,
breaking teeth on its green armour,
holding each other's hands,
licking cloying compliments and complaints
from fingers.

Where is a woman who'd hand you a feast of pears,
split open on a plate surrounded by nuts,
sprinkled with cardamom, dripping with honey?

Discontent

I am still inside this orchard,
whittling on a broken branch,
while she is away to a small dusty town
twenty miles down the road,
where she goes to get the spare parts for the combine,
where our hockey teams raise their fists in winter,

where her cousin Elizabeth is flipping pancakes
for her husband, mute since his stroke.
Heard it from another farmer in the bank.

The chatelaine should be rattling her keys this winter
while I check the cows, tinker with the seeder
for the spring. I should at least finish this year
in some sort of peace. After all,
what could they have to talk about?

Elizabeth on Sacred Stories

Sylva, have you considered the residue of sacred stories?
If you sift carefully between the faded colours,
the leftover hues will teach you how to have a child,
to pay your husband no mind.

Have you thought of the saffron, the blazing reds,
the blue green bushes along the black pool?
Have you gathered blue, the indigo berry
at the beginning of trees thickening around you?
The browns of onion, the green of chamomile.
Greenweed is yellow, and hollyhocks, when dark
provide a most delicate violet.

Stir the putrid liquid in the black waters,
stir briskly the stew of broken stems, roots and leaves,
let them bleed their colours for you.

Pay no mind to the crazy mirrors forever turning,
spinning in moonlight, in sunlight,
spinning you into madness in the pear orchard.

Those stories never are sacred.

Dreams

When you come back, I'd like the smell of yeast high
in a warm kitchen, this is the way I'd like it.
I wander now through the empty room,
see that you left another book
tucked under the *Western Producer*,
and the advertisements for chemical spray.

I don't like your books,
saint books, I'd say, shit books.
I pick up the one about Hildegaard,
rifle through the colour plates,
a blue man, a fiery universe

Hers must be the cuckoo voice
you've played on that choir tape
all day before going off to that woman friend.
I know you turn it off
when I come in to phone for a part,
sell a calf, check on a supplier.

You think I don't hear it out in the barn,
cranked to full volume
disturbing the cows and the CBC.

You dream all day among your jam jars,
I dream at night and will not be told
in the daylight where to sow and reap.

I pick up that book,
the fey Hildegaard of Bingen
now comes to me in the night,
painting a blue universe,
an egg surrounded in yellow flames,
its yolk a pile of small blue eggs.

Banishing me to the pear orchard in my dreams,
a blue tongue unfurls on the eggs.
Does anyone know what this means,
the beginning of a life not found
in the pages of the *Western Producer*?

St. Thomas More

Elizabeth, swollen in a blue gown,
pushes back the wings of her hair,
hands streaked violet with age.
Her child leaps again at his coming.

His merry wit reaches her through the open window
where she sits, winding a skein. Sunlight
falls through the trees behind her
and glints the grey of her hair.

She listens carefully. He speaks of
the lion he married
and of his daughter Meg who spoke Latin
before the king.

She is still cautious. He explains:
Upon leaving the king's court, I cried *boat!*
But you know the London boatmen,
they refused and plunged
their torches into the Thames.

The day is nearly done. He begins walking home,
leaving her on a bed, her hair disheveled.
Her women light candles.

His head is displayed on an iron spike.
She hears witty men in a king's court
bargaining over silver platters and dancing girls.

Her cry escapes, her child leaps.

Thomas Aquinas — Last Words

I.

My wife has packed her amber dress in the trunk up in the attic,
for she is wearing jeans again. It must be the spring
for she comes toward me stranded in this orchard.
I see light and air, the scent of pears and apples reach me
and the crazy mirrors begin to spin again.

This time, small flickerings fade into the sunlight,
the coal heaped shores are now the dark earth,
teeming with insects, worms, delicate green
shoots seek the sun even though they are weeds,
the gold, russet, lime pears
wait, succulent for the harvest.

She holds out to me another book,
the Summa, some ancient book
by some fat monk whose picture
is on the cover and I hear a song
in a man's voice.

II.

Let us go to the fields
where the maiden sleeps,
Solomon's song on a bed of straw.
Let us go, where still she sleeps
before our wedding feast
under sun and moon.

Her white soft belly is private in its growing,
in its humble birthing on the bloody straw.
Let us go, I am ready for my vows,
a rejoicing at my end,
this song of passion
was the Summa, now Solomon's song
on a bed of straw.

Let us go to the fields.

THE FIELDS

"You must be very patient," replied the fox.
"First you will sit down at a little distance
from me, like that in the grass. I shall look at
you out of the corner of my eye, and you will
say nothing."

Antoine de Saint-Exupery
Le Petit Prince

Teach me to hear mermaids singing,
Or to keep off envy's stinging,
And find
What wind
Serves to advance an honest mind.

John Donne
"Song"

Sylva

This body is strange.
The fields are not joyous
nor mysterious as I run through
the pungent stalks on white legs,
my arms flailing over ears of corn.

That night, my master finds me under the bushes,
my red hair shakes over my shoulders.
I avoid his stale wet wool
while he holds the lantern over my face,
exclaims over the rancid breath of the hounds.

Is he my master because he offers me a raw steak?
The blood is high in my nostrils as he tells me
I am a vixen in a woman's body.

After days of following him with obsequious cant,
I wonder as I collapse into a cacophony of vowels
before him, should I give in,

wear this white shift, use a fork,
sleep in his fresh sheeted bed
curled between his head and knees.
Shall I never again gather the bones of a chicken
that I devoured in my own bed?

I sleep.
My master wakes me and I must eat.
Too tired with all this thinking,
this studying of my master, his ways,
his house, his people, his country.
In his synthetic air, I sleep.

My master's eyes are bored.
Vixen, you are deaf,
you are as you always were.

The Fox

A boy from Sparta
hid me under his robe,
letting me eat into him
before I would be discovered
by the guards. He would die
slumped at their feet, my tail
switching out from his cloak.

Now, I am under Sylva's dress,
that brushing sound of my tail
will annoy you, Master. I should become dispersed
in a sea of sound, a civilization of manners,
fine breeding designed to bring
a rousing roar of approval from assemblies
and theatre houses.

To you and the madding crowd,
I am only a portrait, Sylva moving about
in tapestried rooms, sweetly encumbered
by silks and velvets, and long winter days.

In this portrait, she presses me closer
to her womb beneath her amber dress.

The Lure

In my den, I paw my thoughts
before language as if they were fond old tricks.
They are chickens easily devoured,
eggs quickly sucked into my mouth,
farmers outsmarted and hounds
thrown off my scent.

My eyes test the sun
high over my den. I see you eating
a pear, your body swaying
as you tramp through the wheat,
a young, stalwart farmer.
You must have slept in your fields that night
for a tattered blanket flaps around your legs.

You raise your arms to the sun,
and in a fit of merriment,
you adroitly flip onto your back.

Blinking, I emerge.
You are not my husband,
who is still sulking by the black pool,
feeding our hounds,
tinkering with the seeder.

You were in the orchard,
hiding behind the blue black bushes.
I saw you at times, your back disappeared
into the trees, your face a mask against the sun,
a witness to the love between my husband and I,
a divine love, the one that carried me
through the lives of the saints. All that love
is a young farmer whose language
begins with our bodies imprinted on my mind.

Farming Exhibits

There you are, clumping through the art gallery,
jeans, cowboy boots and a straw dusted shirt.
At my insistence, you survey my creations.
With great intensity in my raw voice, I tell you
these are your stories. The farming life,
the sower and the seed, the olive branch.
I've copied the text faithfully,
wouldn't dare change a word, I've gone beyond
language, given them a visual edge.
I've made you famous.

You shift your feet, glance at your watch and the sky.
I rush toward the wall, why won't you tell me more stories?
You could point, mime, gesture,
dance or scribble a few words on a notepad.
Whatever I get from that
will be good enough won't it?

I gotta seed, you say and clump out the door.

Song to the Farmer

My hair once oiled your feet.
You, not I, knew what it meant.

Now you gather me, small and white,
freshly wakened from my sleep.

Please stay.
You are a tent over me,
a canopy of swallows,
and I will quickly embroider
in gold thread,
their resting and mating.

The swallows are startled into flight.
You gather me.
Now we cover the sky.

Glossolalia

Following you like a north star,
I spoke in tongues.
Against the moss on swollen fences
you stand, whittling,
listening to me retell the stories
you taught me.

Stories of the generations before me,
the exotic and the strange
all linked in the glossolalia of the heavens

until in the stillness, the moon
passes over your face. It is expectant.
I am puzzled. What am I to say?

The Sacred Heart

On the edge of the coulee, I stalk your field.
I must have your body again.

How you held me, traveled the universe
in my eyes, my naked body, warm, dark.
You flung open fearlessly, the door
to the richest province of my being,

your broad hands gathering at every stride,
every wild and verdant flower,
the secret varieties, the strange and pungent odours,
random in all their beauty.

I must have your body again,
your gaze most intrepid,
your hands, bold and strong.

I spy your red jacket beckoning from the shade
of your monstrous tractor.
You take my hand and open your coat.
On top of your overalls, you lead my fingers
to a warm, pulsating heart.

I withdraw ever so slightly.
My eyes search over the vastness
of the coulee at my feet.

The Marriage Question

Why don't we get married?
What are earthly husbands for anyway?

I suppress a sneeze
among your wood chips and shavings.
You are shoveling chop into the pail
in your half finished barn,
the wind having swept the old one
away last fall, the splintered planks
are still encrusted in the snow and ice.

You are very helpful and always around.
When I don't have the words, you write them for me.
When I am mute with fear, you offer me your hands.

The silent cattle listen for you
to bring the chop, you stand in the ring,
offer the strands of hay.
Their breath, individual wisps of incense, rise
as they lower their heads into the ring.

Like a priest of Melchizedek of old,
you stand mute.
The mysteries of the flesh come and go,
in and out of the ring, your body bending
with the cows.

I silently wait and watch from a distance,
standing on snow and straw. I am troubled.

There is language between us now.
In the ring of our bodies, we are finally human.
I thought it was such a good idea,
it makes so much sense that two good people
get together, build a life.
You speak, I can sign.

You remain silent, unmoving.
You do not warm to this proposal.
I move closer to the feeding station
with the animals.

Independence

It was you who I loved,
before I caressed the body of my husband,
you, who stood in my mind,
a silent pole on the flat prairie.
I would walk by in later years,
show you the daughter I bore

and you'd shift your feet in shy politeness,
receiving the pain and absurdities
in my soaring hands, in my broken vowels,
the queer pitch of my voice shattering
the spoken tongue.

Your body quivered in my own
throughout the days and nights
in this land of flat and muffled voices.

You fought for me, for us, for our language,
for the word in me while others shook their heads.
You were shunned, you had gone mad, people said.
Somewhere you died, I discovered. Your body
disappeared from a sod shanty no longer than your bones.

These days, I fight alone with the word in me.
Secretly, I think you died for me.

The Fox Wife

After a long day, you've showered off the harvest dust,
I've stored the canning jars in the cellar,
set the frozen steak out to thaw, I must
store the saint books in the attic tomorrow.

You stop at the bedroom door, watch my tail brush out
from the covers, my fine hairs leave a path of red needles
over the white eyelet lace. You've never seen my tail until now,

you've never seen me cavorting in your fields,
disappear into the pungent rows of rape
crushed under your wheel,
nose out a labyrinth etched into the prairie soil.

Envy, too long have I loved you,
admired your portraits, refined your stories,
borrowed your clothes, imitated your speech,
my path was a labyrinth whose green walls

once blocked my return to you, my husband
now aghast at my tail, my upturned nose,
the fiery shock of hair, my small dainty hands
should have warned you

of what I've come to know
what you will soon know,
how I stalk a language of the body,
how I stalk a body most delicious.

Deaf Geography

I am Saskatchewan born,
lovely, dark, twinned with Russia.
My flesh remains on the steppes
in the young colony settling down
for the first winter with a deaf eye
to the cattle, potatoes in the cellar,
children in overalls, boiled home noodles
steaming the windows.

Lovely, I am deaf born,
a fox twinned with the hearing,
a shadow colony settling noiselessly
among these stubborn Russian Germans,
thrift and hard work.

Long ago in Russia,
wolves, dark shadows in the sparse birch
haunted the rich bourgeoisie
frozen inside the turrets of onion roofs.
Lovely, I dart out from the ice crusted homes
out onto the prairies toward the wolves
in dark consent.

Acknowledgements

This book has required a twenty-five year journey, which was something akin to Penelope's weaving by day and undoing it all in the dark of night. I would like to thank all those who have encouraged me as a writer during those long years: the late Anne Szumigalski and Elizabeth Smart, Phyllis Webb, Patrick Lane, Tim Lilburn and, more recently, Jeanette Lynes. Without their encouragement and faith, I would have dismissed my scribbling as resulting from a fevered brain.

Paul Wilson deserves particular mention as an editor with an uncanny sense of direction. His gifts have enabled this manuscript to shine.

I would also like to thank the company of women with whom I journey on a daily basis. Their critique of my writing as well as their thoughts, questions, struggles, and concerns have found their way into this manuscript. I am indebted to my sisters, Ruth Cey, Carol Keller, and my "adopted" sister, Dorene Steele. This list also includes my colleagues from the Regina Public School Board: Sara Randall Nadurak, Gillian Sernich, Cindi Orthner, and Jewel Whyte, who provided encouragement and feedback on various aspects of the manuscript. I also want to thank Dr. Elspeth Tulloch from Laval University for her honest and unflinching eye. Sr. Sarah Doser, FSE, and Sr. Timothy Prokes, SSND in their seminal work on the theology of the body also provided material and insights that sparked the genesis of the entire manuscript. Finally, I wish to thank Marina Kostiuk for her assistance in preparing the manuscript for submission to Hagios Press

I would like to extend my gratitude to the remaining leaders of the Saskatchewan deaf community who are among those in the last generation of a dying deaf community in our province. Their welcome and belief in me, an outsider uninitiated in the richness of their sign language and culture, has enabled me to write this manuscript with their names inscribed in my heart: Bob and Lucille Hutchinson, John and Lydia Storey, Carlyle and Betty Hall, Ed and Vi Dittrick, Roger Schmid, Walter Mason, Ray and Paulette Smith, Janet and Kenneth Dittrick, Mary Jasper, Leslie Dunn, Art Hillcox, Allard Thomas, and Walter and Eunice Markin.

Finally, I would like to thank my husband, Murray, for his uncommon patience, and our daughters, Anna and Paula, for allowing me to quote poetry to them.

Earlier versions of these poems appeared in *Grain*, *The Fiddlehead*, *Contemporary Verse II*, and the anthology, *Heading Out*. "Farming Exhibits" was performed by Roy Challis at an SWG conference in April 2003.

Notes

"The Lie." A sarcophagus is a burial tomb reserved mostly for royalty and nobility. Carved effigies were placed on top of the actual coffin. In case of married couples, the husband and wife would lie side by side, not on top of each other as I have suggested in the poem.

"Christmas Pear 1" — a Christmas tradition in English folklore where a young woman walks backward around a pear tree three times and looks into the branches to discover the face of her true love.

"Geertgen Tot Sint Jans: The Holy Kinship" — a type of portraiture in the late 15th and early 16th centuries called a Holy Kinship, or Holy Company, in which St. Anne and members of her family are present.

"Jan Van Eyck: Giovanni Arnolfini and His Bride." The portrait provides certain documentation for the marriage of Giovanni Arnolfini and Giovanna Cenami in 1434. The bride and groom were children of Italian merchants.

"Chartres" — a gothic cathedral southwest of Paris which has possibly the best rose windows in all of France. Finally completed in 1220, the cathedral required 66 years to build. Chartres is also famous for its labyrinth embedded in the stone floor.

"Book of Hours" — a breviary of prayers for certain times of the day and seasons.

"Annunciation." "Let all mortal flesh keep silence" is taken from the Liturgy of St. James, 4th Century, set to "Picardy," a French carol.

"Rembrandt's Pears." Rembrandt van Rijn (1606-1669), a Dutch artist, never painted pears. The poem is inspired by his painting, "Susanna and the Elders," because of Susanna's obviously pear-shaped body.

"Chatelaine" — term used for the mistress of the medieval household.

"St. Augustine" (354-430) — famous for his *Confessions,* in which he describes his conversion. When elaborating on the sexual sins of his youth, he particularly dwells on the account of raiding a pear orchard with his friends.

"Temptation in the Garden." "Lavendar's Blue" is a nursery rhyme.

"Artifacts." The poem refers to three famous works of art: the ancient pottery found at Knossos, the *Book of Kells* (ca. 800), an illuminated medieval manuscript, and the unicorn tapestry, "A Mon Seul Desir" (late 15th century).

"The Odyssey." Odysseus incurs the wrath of the gods and is forced to undergo a 20-year perilous journey before being allowed to return to his wife, Penelope, in Ithaca. Penelope, on the other hand, weaves by day and undoes her weaving by night in order to outsmart her suitors who would take Odysseus's place. The line, "the works of days and hands," is inspired from Hesiod and is taken directly from T. S. Eliot's "The Love Song of J. Alfred Prufrock."

"The Holy." ". . . holy things are for the holy" is taken from the liturgy of the Ukrainian Catholic Church.

"Boadicea," or Boudicca, was a Celtic queen (ca. 60 AD) who fought against the Romans during their occupation of Britain.

"Simone Weil" — a French mystic and philosopher (1909-43) who is famous for her work, "Waiting for God."

"Catherine Earnshaw" is the heroine of *Wuthering Heights* (Emily Brontë, 1818-48), trapped in an obsessive love affair with Heathcliff.

"Isolde the Fair to Evelyn Waugh (*Brideshead Revisited*)." The poem is a juxtaposition of two literary works, the myth of Tristan and Isolde (predating Arthurian legends), a story of two doomed lovers, and Evelyn Waugh's novel, *Brideshead Revisited*, which chronicles a doomed love affair. The phrase, "cloak random and wild," is from Joseph Bedier's translation of the myth from the French.

"Ezekial 16" — an Old Testament prophet who compares the love of God for a fickle generation to a husband's love for an unfaithful wife.

"Fanny Mendelssohn: A Letter to Felix." Fanny (1805-47) composed music which was, at times, of better quality than that of her famous brother, Felix. He claimed some of her music as his own.

"Marie Curie" (1867-91) discovered radium with her husband, Pierre. Renoir was an impressionist painter in Paris about that time.

"Augustine's Pear." "Late have I loved You, beauty so ancient yet so new" is from St. Augustine's *Confessions*.

"Noise." " . . . a holy fire, sizzling" is inspired by St. Augustine's *Confessions*, where he writes, "and all around me in my ears were the sizzling and frying of unholy loves."

"Renoir: On the Terrace." This portrait of two sisters in the impressionist style is presented as mother and daughter in the poem.

"Lara: To Zhivago" was inspired by Pasternak's novel of a doctor engaged in a love affair against the backdrop of the Russian Revolution.

"Karensgaard" is the name of a Danish farm. I merely liked the name.

"George Sand." The relationship between George Sand (1804-76) and Chopin (1810-49) was, at best, turbulent. She never had a child by Chopin as suggested by the poem.

"Héloïse" (1101-62) was seduced by Abelard (1079-1142), a tutor in the house of her uncle in Paris. She became pregnant with their child, whom she named Astrolabe. Abelard, who was castrated by order of her uncle, insisted that Héloïse join a religious order. He went on to become one of the major philosophers of the 13th century. Héloïse became a prioress at her abbey.

"Teresa of Avila," a Spanish mystic (1515-82), was known for her extreme common sense and her intense mystical experiences.

"Pieta" was inspired by Michelangelo's *Pieta* (1498-99) which is now housed in St. Peter's Basilica in Rome. The statue depicts Mary holding the body of her son following the crucifixion.

"Dorothy Day: Annunciation." Dorothy Day (1897-1980) is a candidate for canonization in the Catholic Church. She was known for her political activism on the behalf of poor workers in New York City in the 1930s. She and Peter Maurin founded the Catholic Worker Movement in 1933. Her conversion to Catholicism occurred after the birth of her daughter, and resulted in her being rejected by her common-law partner, who was a scientist.

"Silence." Zechariah is the husband of Elizabeth, who was the cousin of Mary, mother of Jesus. He was struck dumb in the temple when informed by the angel that his aged wife was about to bear a child.

"Dreams." Hildegaard of Bingen (1098-1179) is known for her visionary writings, which include the pollution of the earth in later centuries. Many of her works celebrate sexuality, fertility, and the "greening" of the earth. She also composed music.

"St. Thomas More" (1478-1535) was a lawyer in the Tudor court, and was executed by King Henry VIII for not agreeing to support his move to separate from the Roman Catholic Church in order to establish himself as the head of the church in England. Henry needed a pretext to divorce his Catholic wife in order to marry Anne Boelyn.

"Thomas Aquinas" (1225-74) is best known for his *Summa*, a gargantuan synthesis of Aristotelian philosophy and church teachings. Upon completion of his work, he had a vision which convinced him that all he had written amounted to "straw."

"Sylva" was inspired by Jean Vercors's novel *Sylva*, a fantastical tale of a man who attempts to tame a woman who is really a fox.

"The Fox" is modeled on the story of the Spartan boy who captures a live fox, intending to eat it. He hides the fox under his cloak in order to escape detection by soldiers who confront the boy with his illicit action. In order to maintain his denial, the boy allows the fox to chew his innards while displaying no emotion.

"Glossolalia." The term denotes the singing or speaking in "tongues" which is the ability to speak in several languages without any foreknowledge of them.

"The Marriage Question." Melchisidek represents a line of priests in the Old Testament.

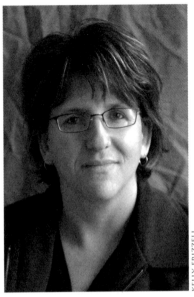

KELLY FRIZZELL

Joanne Weber earned a BA honours in English literature at the University of Saskatchewan and a master's degree in Library Science from the University of Alberta. After receiving a BEd from the University of Saskatchewan, she did graduate work at Gallaudet University in Washington, DC. Joanne is a resource room teacher in the Deaf and Hard of Hearing Program at Thom Collegiate in Regina, Saskatchewan. Fluent in American Sign Language, she has been involved with the deaf community in leadership roles at local and provincial levels. Joanne and her husband live in Regina with their two teenage daughters.